COMPLETE GUIDE TO UNDERSTANDING LASIK EYE SURGERY

Everything You Need To Know About Laser Vision, Procedure Steps, Recovery, Risks, Benefits, Costs, For Perfect Sight Enhancement

KLEIN HOYLE

© [KLEIN HOYLE] [2024]

All rights reserved.

No part of this book may be reproduced, distributed, or transmitted in any form or by any means, including photocopying, recording, or other electronic or mechanical methods, without the publisher's prior written permission, with the exception of brief quotations in critical reviews and certain other noncommercial uses permitted by copyright law.

Disclaimer

The content in this book is based on the author's expertise and comprehension of the topic. The author has no affiliation or link with any corporation, business, or person. This book is meant to give general information and educational material only, and it should not be interpreted as professional medical advice. Always seek the advice of a skilled healthcare expert if you have any queries about medical issues or treatments. The author and publisher expressly disclaim any responsibility resulting directly or indirectly from the use or use of the information included in this book.

Table of Contents

CHAPTER 1 9
- Introduction To LASIK Eye Surgery.................9
- Definition And Overview Of LASIK 9
- History And Development Of The Procedure 10
- Benefits Of Lasik Surgery............................11
  - 1. Improved eyesight: 11
  - 2. Quick Recovery:...................................12
  - 3. Long-Term Results: 12
  - 4. Convenience and Comfort: 12
  - 5. Cost Savings: 12
- Common Myths And Misconceptions..............13
  - 1. Myth: Lasik is painful...........................13
  - 2. Myth: LASIK Results Are Temporary........13
  - 3. Myth: LASIK may cause blindness............14
  - 4. Myth: LASIK Is Only for Young People 14
  - 5. Myth: LASIK isn't safe since it is new. 14

CHAPTER 2 17
- How Does The Eye Work? 17
- Basic Anatomy Of The Eye..........................17
- How Vision Works.....................................18

Common Vision Problems Corrected By LASIK 19

The Role Of The Cornea In Vision 20

CHAPTER 3 23

Eligibility For LASIK Surgery 23

Eligibility Criteria For Lasik..........................23

Medical Conditions That Can Affect Candidacy 25

Age Considerations 27

Importance Of A Comprehensive Eye Exam 29

CHAPTER 4 31

Preoperative Preparations 31

Initial Consultation And Evaluation 31

Pre-Surgical Eye Care Tips 32

   1. Avoid Contact Lenses:............................32

   2. Keep Your Eyes Hydrated: 32

   3. Protect Your Eyes: 33

   4. Follow Medication Instructions: 33

Instructions For The Day Before Surgery..........33

   1. Avoid Makeup and Lotions: 33

   2. Arrange Transportation: 34

   3. Follow Fasting Instructions: 34

   4. Obtain Plenty of Rest: 34

What To Expect On The Day Of Surgery? 34
    1. Arrival and Paperwork: 35
    2. Pre-Operative Preparation: 35
    3. The Procedure: 35
    4. Post-Operative Care: 35

CHAPTER 5 37
    The Lasik Procedure 37
    Step-By-Step Explanation Of The LASIK Technique 37
        1. Preparation: 37
        3. Reshaping the Cornea: 38
        4. Flap Replacement: 38
        5. Post-operative Care: 38
        6. Follow-up Visits: 38
    Types Of LASIK Procedures (For Example, Bladeless LASIK, Classic LASIK) 39
    The Role Of The Surgeon And Surgical Team....41
        1. Surgeon: 41
        2. Surgical Team: 41
    Duration And What To Expect During The Procedure 42

    1. Preparation: 42

    2. Surgery: 43

    3. LASIK operation: 43

    4. Post-operative Care: 43

    5. Follow-up Visits: 44

CHAPTER 6 45

Postoperative Care And Recovery 45

Immediate Post-Surgical Care Instructions 45

    Rest and relax: 45

    Eye Protection: 46

    Use Prescribed Eye drops: 46

    Avoid Rubbing Your Eyes. 46

    Follow-up Appointment: 47

Timeline Of Recovery And Healing 47

    Immediate Recovery: 47

    First week: 47

    Two to four weeks. 48

    Long-term Recovery: 48

Managing Discomfort And Side Effects 49

    Dry eyes: 49

    Light Sensitivity: 49

    Halos or glare: 50
    Discomfort: 50
  Follow-Up Appointments And Long-Term Care 50
    First Post-Operation Visit: 51
    Subsequent visits: 51
    Long-term Care: 51
CHAPTER 7 53
  Risks And Complications 53
  Common Dangers Related To LASIK 53
  Potential Issues And How They Are Handled 54
    1. Infection: 55
    2. Glare or halos: 55
    4. Regression: 56
  Long-Term Hazards And Uncommon
  Consequences 56
    1. Dry eye syndrome: 56
    2. Vision changes: 56
    3. Corneal thinning: 57
    4. Complications of enhancement operations: . 57
  How To Reduce Risks And Achieve A Favorable
  Result 58

1. Choosing a competent physician: 58

2. Following pre-operative instructions: 58

3. Disclosing medical history and risk factors: . 59

4. Awareness of the technique and the dangers: 59

CHAPTER 8 61

Alternatives To Lasik 61

Other Refractive Surgeries 61

Nonsurgical Options 63

Comparing LASIK To Other Vision Correction Methods 64

Choosing The Best Option For Your Needs 65

CHAPTER 9 67

Cost And Insurance Considerations 67

Typical Prices For LASIK Surgery 67

Factors That Impact Costs 68

Insurance Coverage And Financing Alternatives 70

How To Analyze And Choose A LASIK Provider 71

1. Experience and expertise: 71

3. Reputation and reviews: 72

4. Appointment process: 72

CHAPTER 10 75

Advancements In LASIK Technology...............75

Latest Innovations In LASIK Technology 75

Custom LASIK And Wavefront-Guided Procedures 76

The Future Of LASIK: Emerging Trends 78

How Technology Improves Results And Safety ..79

Conclusion 82

THE END 85

ABOUT THIS BOOK

The "Complete Guide to Understanding LASIK Eye Surgery" is an invaluable resource for anybody contemplating LASIK, providing a thorough review of the surgery and its numerous elements. This book opens with an overview of LASIK, offering a clear explanation and tracking its historical evolution. Readers will receive insight into the many advantages of LASIK, which vary from enhanced vision to increased convenience, while also refuting prevalent myths and misunderstandings about this operation.

Understanding how the eye works is critical to understanding the mechanics of LASIK. This tutorial examines the fundamental anatomy of the eye and explains how vision works. It focuses on common vision disorders including myopia, hyperopia, and astigmatism, all of which may be corrected by LASIK. The cornea's significance in vision is stressed, demonstrating why its reshaping is so important in the LASIK treatment.

Determining suitability for LASIK is an important step, and this book explains the main eligibility requirements. It highlights numerous medical issues that may impact a person's fitness for surgery, as well as the significance of age. The need for a full eye exam is emphasized, ensuring that prospective patients realize the necessity for a thorough screening before advancing.

Pre-operative preparations are well explained, bringing readers through the first consultation and assessment procedure. This book offers realistic pre-surgical eye care advice and specifics about what to anticipate the day before and the day of surgery, preparing patients for a seamless experience.

The guide's main focus is a thorough, step-by-step explanation of the LASIK technique. It delves into several LASIK procedures, including classic and bladeless approaches, and clarifies the duties of the surgeon and surgical team. The length of the treatment and what patients may anticipate throughout the surgery are clearly defined, demystifying the process.

Post-operative care and recuperation are critical to attaining the greatest results. This guide provides immediate post-surgery care instructions and a recovery and healing timeframe. It offers tips for dealing with pain and probable side effects, stressing the significance of follow-up visits and long-term care to achieve long-term outcomes.

Risks and problems are unavoidable concerns, and this book discusses them candidly. It covers the typical dangers involved with LASIK, as well as possible problems and how to handle them. Long-term hazards and unusual problems are also covered, along with measures for reducing these risks and increasing the possibility of a good result.

For individuals considering alternative treatments, This book compares LASIK to other refractive operations like as PRK, LASEK, and SMILE, as well as non-surgical alternatives such as glasses and contact lenses. This comparison enables readers to make more educated judgments regarding the best vision correction treatment for their circumstances.

Cost and insurance issues are realistic elements that should not be ignored. This article discusses the usual expenses of LASIK surgery, the variables that influence these prices, and the available insurance coverage and financing alternatives. Tips for assessing and selecting a LASIK provider guarantee that readers discover a reliable and appropriate facility.

Finally, this book discusses the most recent breakthroughs in LASIK technology, including bespoke LASIK and wave front-guided surgeries. It examines developing trends and the future of LASIK, emphasizing how technology developments enhance patient results and safety.

In conclusion, "Complete Guide to Understanding LASIK Eye Surgery" is a useful, detailed, and engaging resource that covers all aspects of LASIK, from the initial decision-making process to the most recent technological advancements, ensuring that readers are well-informed and prepared for their vision correction journey.

CHAPTER 1

Introduction To LASIK Eye Surgery

Definition And Overview Of LASIK

LASIK, or Laser-Assisted In Situ Keratomileusis, is a popular and very efficient surgical technique used to repair common visual issues such as myopia (nearsightedness), hyperopia (farsightedness), and astigmatism. The technique involves using a specialized laser to reshape the cornea, the transparent front section of the eye, enabling light entering the eye to be correctly focused on the retina, resulting in sharper vision.

The technique normally consists of three steps: generating a thin flap on the cornea, altering the underlying corneal tissue using an excimer laser, and repositioning the corneal flap. The whole procedure is rather short, sometimes requiring 10 to 15 minutes for each eye, and is done as an outpatient, which means patients may go home the same day.

History And Development Of The Procedure

The evolution of LASIK eye surgery is a remarkable story of scientific and medical progress. The idea of utilizing a laser to reshape the cornea goes back to the 1970s. The early work was based on the theory of keratomileusis, which involves freezing and physically shaping the cornea. However, this procedure was not very exact and posed major hazards.

The advent of the excimer laser, which could accurately remove minuscule quantities of tissue without injuring the surrounding regions, was a watershed moment in the 1980s. Dr. Ioannis Pallikaris, a Greek ophthalmologist, conducted the first LASIK operation in 1989, using an excimer laser and a corneal flap. This was an important milestone in refractive surgery.

Throughout the 1990s and early 2000s, advances in technology and surgical procedures helped to increase the safety and efficacy of LASIK. The use of wavefront-guided LASIK and femtosecond lasers to create the corneal flap improved the procedure's accuracy and results. Today, LASIK is one of the most popular elective operations in the world, with millions of patients benefiting from considerable vision improvements.

Benefits Of Lasik Surgery

LASIK surgery has various advantages that make it an appealing alternative for anyone looking to lessen or remove their reliance on glasses or contact lenses.

1. **Improved eyesight:** The major advantage of LASIK is considerable improvement in eyesight. Most patients acquire 20/20 vision or greater, enabling them to carry out regular activities without the need for corrective glasses.

2. Quick Recovery: One of the advantages of LASIK is the comparatively short recovery period. Many patients notice better eyesight almost immediately following the surgery, and most may resume regular activities within a day or two.

3. Long-Term Results: LASIK corrects eyesight for the long term. While certain age-related changes in eyesight may occur over time, LASIK outcomes are often stable and may endure for many years.

4. Convenience and Comfort: LASIK removes the hassle and discomfort that comes with wearing glasses or contact lenses. Patients no longer have to be concerned about cleaning and maintaining contact lenses or dealing with damaged or missing glasses.

5. Cost Savings: While the initial cost of LASIK may be high, surgery can result in long-term cost savings by lowering or eliminating the need for prescription eyeglasses and contact lenses.

6. Improved Quality of Life: Better eyesight may have a significant influence on a person's quality of life. It may improve athletic performance, driving ability, and general well-being.

Common Myths And Misconceptions

Despite its popularity and proven efficacy, LASIK surgery is plagued by myths and misunderstandings. Addressing these may assist prospective candidates to make educated judgments regarding the procedure:

1. Myth: Lasik is painful.

LASIK is often painless. Numbing eye drops are utilized to keep the patient comfortable during the treatment. Some patients may suffer moderate soreness or a gritty sensation after surgery, although this usually resolves within a few hours.

2. Myth: LASIK Results Are Temporary.
LASIK outcomes are supposed to be permanent. While natural aging may impair eyesight over time,

the structural alterations performed to the cornea during LASIK are permanent.

3. Myth: LASIK may cause blindness.

The risk of serious consequences following LASIK, including blindness, is exceedingly minimal. LASIK is regarded as one of the safest elective operations, with a high success rate.

4. Myth: LASIK Is Only for Young People

LASIK is frequently done on individuals in their 20s to 40s, but it may also benefit older persons who satisfy the appropriate health and visual conditions. Age is not a disqualifying criterion.

5. Myth: LASIK isn't safe since it is new.

LASIK has a long history of safety and effectiveness, dating back over 30 years. Technology has improved and advanced throughout time, making it safer.

Understanding these facts may help eliminate anxieties and misunderstandings about LASIK, enabling people to approach the treatment with more confidence and clarity.

CHAPTER 2

How Does The Eye Work?

Basic Anatomy Of The Eye

Understanding the fundamentals of how our eyes work is critical before undergoing LASIK surgery. The eye is a wonder of biological engineering, consisting of several sophisticated elements that operate in tandem to give humans vision. The eye is made up of the cornea, iris, pupil, lens, retina, and optic nerve.

The cornea is the translucent covering that protects the front of the eye. It serves as a protective barrier while also playing an important function in focusing light on the retina. The iris, the colorful component of the eye, governs the size of the pupil, which determines how much light enters the eye.

The lens, located behind the iris and pupil, directs light onto the retina. The retina, situated in the back of the eye, contains millions of light-sensitive cells known as rods and cones. These cells convert light into electrical impulses that are sent to the brain via the optic nerve.

Understanding this fundamental anatomy sets the groundwork for understanding how LASIK surgery works and why it helps treat vision difficulties.

How Vision Works

Vision is a multi-step process that begins with the admission of light into the eye. Light enters the eye via the cornea and is refracted, or twisted, to concentrate on the retina. The lens then changes the focus to guarantee a crisp picture.

When light enters the retina, it is absorbed by the rods and cones and converted into electrical impulses. These impulses are subsequently carried by the optic nerve to the brain, where they are processed as visual pictures.

This process occurs rapidly and is responsible for our capacity to perceive the world around us. However, anomalies in the shape of the cornea or the length of the eyeball may cause visual issues such as myopia (nearsightedness), hyperopia (farsightedness), and astigmatism.

Common Vision Problems Corrected By LASIK

LASIK surgery is a common treatment for treating a variety of visual issues, including myopia, hyperopia, and astigmatism. Myopia develops when the eyeball is excessively long or the cornea is too steep, making distant things look hazy. Hyperopia, on the other hand, happens when the eyeball is too short or the cornea is excessively flat, resulting in blurred close-up images.

Astigmatism occurs when the cornea or lens has an uneven shape, resulting in distorted or blurred vision at all distances. LASIK surgery may efficiently cure these visual issues by reshaping the cornea, enabling light to concentrate correctly on the retina.

Individuals may assess if LASIK surgery is right for them by learning the specifics of their visual condition.

The Role Of The Cornea In Vision

The cornea is the outermost lens of the eye and plays an important role in vision. It refracts light and directs it to the retina, where visual pictures are produced. The shape and curvature of the cornea are critical to preserving good eyesight.

Individuals with vision difficulties such as myopia, hyperopia, or astigmatism have an uneven cornea, which causes light to concentrate incorrectly on the retina.

LASIK surgery corrects this imperfection by reshaping the cornea, resulting in enhanced vision without the need for corrective glasses.

Understanding the function of the cornea emphasizes the need for accurate reshaping during LASIK surgery and explains why it is such an effective therapy for a wide range of vision issues.

CHAPTER 3

Eligibility For LASIK Surgery

Eligibility Criteria For Lasik

When contemplating LASIK surgery, one of the first stages is to see whether you are a good candidate. LASIK isn't for everyone, but technological breakthroughs have increased the number of prospective candidates. In general, you must be older than 18, have had stable eyesight for at least a year, and have healthy corneas. However, there are more characteristics to examine.

First and foremost, your eye prescription is important. LASIK may cure nearsightedness, farsightedness, and astigmatism, but the severity of your prescription is important. Extreme prescriptions may not be appropriate for LASIK, but alternative vision correction treatments may be a possibility. Your eye doctor will evaluate your prescription and decide if LASIK is right for you.

Furthermore, the thickness of your cornea is crucial. LASIK reshapes the cornea to correct vision, hence enough corneal thickness is required for the surgery. If your corneas are excessively thin, alternative vision correction techniques may be advised instead.

Your general eye health is another consideration. Dry eye syndrome, glaucoma, and cataracts are all conditions that may impair your eligibility for LASIK. These disorders may influence the procedure's outcome and offer dangers throughout the healing phase. Your eye doctor will assess your eye health and decide if LASIK is appropriate for you.

Pregnancy and certain drugs may potentially influence LASIK candidacy. Hormonal changes during pregnancy might temporarily affect eyesight, necessitating a postpartum treatment. Some drugs, including steroids, might impair recovery and may prevent you from having LASIK until you have stopped taking them for a set length of time.

Overall, the qualifying requirements for LASIK include age, prescription, corneal thickness, and overall eye health. A thorough consultation by a skilled eye surgeon will evaluate if LASIK is the best option for you.

Medical Conditions That Can Affect Candidacy

Certain medical issues may affect your eligibility for the LASIK procedure. While LASIK is a safe and successful surgery for many individuals, it may not be appropriate for those who have specific medical conditions. To establish if LASIK is a suitable choice for you, you must first address any medical issues you may have with your eye doctor.

Autoimmune diseases are a prevalent issue that might impact LASIK's candidacy. Conditions including rheumatoid arthritis, lupus, and Sjogren's syndrome may impair the body's capacity to recover effectively. Because LASIK includes reshaping the cornea, adequate healing is essential for a positive result. Individuals with autoimmune illnesses may be more likely to have problems or delayed healing after LASIK.

Similarly, diabetics may experience difficulties with LASIK candidacy. Diabetes may damage the blood vessels in the eyes, raising the risk of problems including diabetic retinopathy. Furthermore, diabetes might impair recovery, which is critical for the effectiveness of LASIK surgery. Your eye doctor will assess your diabetes control and general eye health to decide if LASIK is appropriate for you.

Chronic dry eye syndrome, glaucoma, and cataracts are among the medical issues that might impair LASIK candidacy.

These disorders may influence the procedure's outcome and offer dangers throughout the healing phase. To decide if LASIK is the best option for you, your eye doctor will review your medical history and conduct a thorough eye exam.

Be upfront and honest with your eye doctor about any medical issues you may have. They will give individualized suggestions based on your specific health requirements, allowing you to make an educated choice regarding LASIK surgery.

Age Considerations

When deciding on LASIK candidacy, age is an essential consideration. While LASIK is often suggested for individuals over the age of 18, there is no maximum age for the treatment. However, some age-related changes in the eyes may limit the efficacy of LASIK for older persons.

Young individuals under the age of 18 are typically not considered appropriate candidates for LASIK surgery since their eyes are still growing. LASIK requires vision stability, and younger people's prescriptions may alter as their eyes mature. Before undergoing LASIK surgery, it is suggested that you wait at least a year for your eyesight to settle.

For older persons, age-related changes like as presbyopia may influence LASIK candidacy. Presbyopia is a disorder that impairs near eyesight and often appears around the age of 40. LASIK may correct distant vision, but not presbyopia. However, techniques like as monovision LASIK or multifocal lenses may be suitable for both far and close vision.

Overall, age does not prohibit someone from having a LASIK procedure. Instead, evaluate aspects including eyesight stability, general eye health, and any age-related changes that might alter the procedure's result. Your eye doctor will evaluate your specific circumstances and advise you on whether LASIK is the best option for you at any age.

Importance Of A Comprehensive Eye Exam

A full eye examination is required before LASIK surgery. This exam gives important information about your eye health and helps you decide whether LASIK is best for you. During the examination, your eye doctor will assess many elements of your eyesight and eye health.

First, your eye doctor will determine your refractive error, which might include nearsightedness, farsightedness, and astigmatism. They will assess the curvature of your cornea and the thickness of your corneal tissue to establish the best treatment option for your vision correction.

Your eye doctor will also assess the general health of your eyes. They will look for problems including dry eye syndrome, glaucoma, and cataracts that might influence your eligibility for LASIK surgery. They will also evaluate the stability of your eyesight to verify that LASIK is an appropriate choice for you.

A thorough eye exam may also involve tests like pupil dilation, which enables your doctor to examine the retina and optic nerve more carefully. These tests give important information about the health of your eyes and contribute to the effectiveness of LASIK surgery.

Overall, a complete eye exam is a necessary stage in the LASIK procedure. It enables your eye doctor to evaluate your eye health, decide if LASIK is the best option for you, and create a customized treatment plan to help you accomplish your vision correction objectives. A comprehensive assessment will guarantee a safe and effective LASIK treatment.

CHAPTER 4

Preoperative Preparations

Initial Consultation And Evaluation

Before proceeding with LASIK surgery, you will need to complete an initial consultation and examination. This is your chance to visit with an eye care specialist who will determine whether LASIK is a good fit for you. This session will include a thorough eye examination. This exam may include tests to measure your eye's refractive error, corneal thickness, pupil size, and general eye health. Your medical history and current medicines will also be evaluated to verify that LASIK is safe for you.

The assessment is more than simply assessing if you are a candidate for LASIK; it also involves setting reasonable expectations. Your eye doctor will explain what results you may expect depending on your specific circumstances. They will explain the risks and advantages of LASIK, giving you all the information you need to make an educated choice.

Pre-Surgical Eye Care Tips

Take care of your eyes in the days leading up to your LASIK procedure. Your eye care physician will most likely give you specific instructions based on your circumstances, but here are some basic guidelines to follow:

1. Avoid Contact Lenses: If you use contact lenses, you will most likely need to transition to glasses before surgery. Contact lenses might temporarily alter the curvature of your cornea, thus influencing the accuracy of pre-operative measurements.

2. Keep Your Eyes Hydrated: Dry eyes may be painful and slow the healing process after LASIK. Drink lots of water to stay hydrated, and use lubricating eye drops as required.

3. Protect Your Eyes: Avoid activities that might injure your eyes, such as swimming in chlorine pools or participating in contact sports where you may be struck in the eye.

4. Follow Medication Instructions: If your eye doctor has given any medicines or eye drops, be sure you take them as recommended before surgery.

Instructions For The Day Before Surgery

As your LASIK surgery date approaches, you will be given precise instructions to follow the day before the operation. These guidelines are intended to ensure that everything runs well on the day of surgery. Here's what you may expect:

1. Avoid Makeup and Lotions: On the day of surgery, avoid wearing makeup, lotions, or creams around your eyes. These products may raise the risk of infection during surgery.

2. Arrange Transportation: Because you will most likely be given a sedative to rest during the surgery, you will need someone to transport you home afterward. Arrange transportation ahead of time so you don't have to worry about it on the day of operation.

3. Follow Fasting Instructions: Depending on the kind of anesthetic used during LASIK, you may need to fast for some time before the surgery. Follow your eye care provider's eating and drinking guidelines.

4. Obtain Plenty of Rest: Aim to obtain a decent night's sleep before your LASIK procedure. Being well-rested might make you more peaceful and comfortable throughout the operation.

What To Expect On The Day Of Surgery?

Finally, the big day is here! Here's what you should anticipate on the day of your LASIK surgery:

1. **Arrival and Paperwork:** When you arrive at the LASIK clinic, you will most likely need to fill out some paperwork and supply any required payment information.

2. **Pre-Operative Preparation:** Before the operation, you will go through certain pre-operative procedures. This may involve numbing eye medications to prevent pain during the surgery.

3. **The Procedure:** LASIK surgery usually takes just around 15 minutes for each eye. During the process, you will recline on a comfy bed while a tiny gadget holds your eyes open. Your eye surgeon will use a laser to reshape your cornea and correct your eyesight.

4. **Post-Operative Care:** Following the procedure, you will spend some time in a recovery room. Your eye care team will provide you with post-operative instructions, including how to utilize any prescription drugs or eye drops.

You'll be well-prepared for your LASIK procedure if you follow these pre-operative steps and understand what to anticipate on the day of surgery. Remember to ask any questions you may have at your first appointment and throughout the process to ensure you are comfortable and well-informed.

CHAPTER 5

The Lasik Procedure

Step-By-Step Explanation Of The LASIK Technique

LASIK, or Laser-Assisted In Situ Keratomileusis, is a precise surgical treatment used to correct refractive problems such as nearsightedness, farsightedness, and astigmatism. Here's a step-by-step explanation of what occurs during a LASIK procedure:

1. **Preparation:** Before the operation, your eye surgeon will prescribe numbing eye drops to keep you comfortable throughout. Your eyes will be cleaned, and your eyelids will be held open using a device known as a lid speculum.

2. The surgeon will use either a microkeratome (a precision surgical device with an oscillating blade) or a femtosecond laser to form a thin, hinged flap in the

cornea. This flap provides access to the underlying corneal tissue for reshaping.

3. Reshaping the Cornea: After the corneal flap is raised, a specialized excimer laser is utilized to precisely reshape the cornea depending on your refractive defect. This reshaping procedure is suited to your eye's specific shape and prescription.

4. Flap Replacement: After the cornea has been reshaped, the surgeon carefully repositions the corneal flap to its original position. The cornea's self-adhesive qualities allow the flap to attach spontaneously without the need for sutures.

5. Post-operative Care: Following the surgery, your eyes may feel itchy or dry. Your surgeon will advise you on post-operative care, which may include using prescription eye drops to aid healing and alleviate pain.

6. Follow-up Visits: It is critical to plan follow-up sessions with your eye surgeon to check your healing process and ensure the best visual results. During these sessions, your surgeon will evaluate your eyesight and discuss any concerns you may have.

Throughout the LASIK treatment, modern technologies and thorough surgical procedures are used to deliver accurate outcomes while reducing the potential for problems. While the prospect of having eye surgery may sound scary, LASIK is a safe and successful technique that has helped millions of individuals get sharper vision and minimize their reliance on glasses or contact lenses.

Types Of LASIK Procedures (For Example, Bladeless LASIK, Classic LASIK)

LASIK procedures have changed over time, giving patients more choices and better results. Traditional and bladeless LASIK are the two most frequent forms of LASIK procedures:

1. Traditional LASIK uses a microkeratome, a portable surgical tool with an oscillating blade, to generate the corneal flap. While this treatment has been used effectively for many years and remains popular, some patients may be concerned about the blade's accuracy.

2. Bladeless LASIK, also known as all-laser LASIK, uses a femtosecond laser to generate the corneal flap rather than a microkeratome. This improved laser technique enables a more accurate and adjustable flap production procedure, thereby lowering the risk of flap problems while enhancing visual results.

Both classic LASIK and bladeless LASIK are excellent treatments for treating refractive defects, and the decision between the two may be influenced by variables such as your unique eye anatomy, physician preference, and technical developments available at the surgery facility.

The Role Of The Surgeon And Surgical Team

The effectiveness of a LASIK operation is mainly dependent on the surgeon's ability and the help of a professional surgical team. Here is a summary of the roles they play:

1. Surgeon: The eye surgeon is in charge of completing the LASIK operation with precision and accuracy. Before the procedure, the surgeon will assess your eye health, discuss your objectives and expectations, and establish if you are a good candidate for LASIK. The surgeon supervises each stage of the process, from producing the corneal flap to reshaping the cornea, to provide the best possible results.

2. Surgical Team: Trained experts support the surgeon before, during, and after the LASIK surgery. This team may comprise nurses, surgical technologists, and ophthalmic assistants who collaborate to keep the surgical environment clean, the equipment calibrated correctly, and the patient comfortable and informed during the procedure.

Collaboration and communication between the surgeon and the surgical team are required for a smooth and effective LASIK treatment. Each member plays an important role in providing safe and effective treatment to patients undergoing LASIK surgery.

Duration And What To Expect During The Procedure

A LASIK treatment normally takes 15 to 30 minutes per eye, however, the actual surgical time may vary based on individual characteristics and the intricacy of the case. Here's what to anticipate during the procedure:

1. Preparation: Before the procedure, you will have a complete eye examination to determine your suitability for LASIK. Once you have been approved for the treatment, you will be given information on pre-operative care and any precautions you need take before to surgery.

2. Surgery: When you arrive at the surgical facility for your LASIK surgery, you will be welcomed by the surgical team. After checking in, you'll be prepared for surgery, which will involve numbing eye drops and a comfortable posture on the operating table.

3. LASIK operation: The surgeon will walk you through each phase of the operation, explaining what to anticipate and guaranteeing your comfort throughout. The corneal flap is created and reshaped with accuracy and efficiency, using sophisticated technology and surgical procedures.

4. Post-operative Care: After the LASIK surgery, you will relax momentarily in a recovery area while the surgical team examines your immediate post-operative status. Once the surgeon has cleared you, you will be given post-operative instructions, including how to use prescription eye drops and any activity limitations.

5. Follow-up Visits: It is critical to plan follow-up sessions with your eye surgeon to check your healing process and ensure the best visual results. Your surgeon will evaluate your eyesight, discuss any concerns you may have, and advise you on long-term eye health care.

Overall, LASIK surgery is a fast and simple outpatient treatment that provides many patients with life-changing advantages. With good pre-operative planning, skillful surgical execution, and careful post-operative care, LASIK may offer long-term vision correction and enhance quality of life.

CHAPTER 6

Postoperative Care And Recovery

Immediate Post-Surgical Care Instructions

Following LASIK eye surgery, it is critical to carefully follow initial post-operative care recommendations to guarantee adequate healing and reduce the chance of problems. Your eye surgeon will offer you thorough advice geared to your unique condition, but here are some broad directions you should expect:

Rest and relax:

Rest your eyes right after the operation. Avoid intensive activities like reading, watching television, or using technological gadgets. Give your eyes plenty of rest while they recuperate from surgery.

Eye Protection:

Your surgeon may give you special goggles or shields to wear soon after surgery. These protect your eyes from inadvertent rubbing or bumping, which might disrupt the healing process. Wear them as directed, particularly when sleeping.

Use Prescribed Eye drops:

You'll most likely be given a regimen of eye drops to take after the procedure. These drops help prevent infection, decrease inflammation, and keep your eyes moist while they recover. Follow the dosing directions carefully and use exactly as instructed.

Avoid Rubbing Your Eyes.

Resist the impulse to rub or touch your eyes, since this might displace the corneal flap generated during LASIK surgery and cause difficulties. If your eyes are itching or inflamed, use artificial tears to soothe them.

Follow-up Appointment:

Schedule a follow-up visit with your eye surgeon for the day after your operation. During this session, your surgeon will inspect your eyes to verify normal healing and answer any questions or concerns you may have.

Timeline Of Recovery And Healing

The healing scheduled for LASIK surgery might vary from person to person, but here's a broad outline of what to expect:

Immediate Recovery:

Immediately after surgery, your eyesight may be cloudy or fuzzy, and you may feel pain or irritation. This is typical and should improve during the first few hours or days after the treatment.

First week:
During the first week after recuperation, your eyesight may improve gradually as your eyes mend. During

this period, you may continue to suffer visual changes, dryness, or light sensitivity.

Two to four weeks.

By the end of the first month, most patients have significantly improved their eyesight and can resume routine activities. However, it is critical to continue taking the prescription eye drops as advised and to schedule follow-up consultations with your eye surgeon.

Long-term Recovery:

While you may see instant improvements in your vision after LASIK surgery, it might take many months for your eyes to settle and achieve their peak clarity. Be patient, and continue to follow your surgeon's post-operative recommendations.

Managing Discomfort And Side Effects

While LASIK surgery is typically safe and successful, it is common to have some pain and side effects throughout the healing period. Here are some recommendations for addressing frequent issues:

Dry eyes:

Many individuals have transient dryness or discomfort in their eyes after LASIK surgery. To keep your eyes moist and pleasant, use artificial tears as prescribed by your surgeon. Avoiding dry surroundings, such as air-conditioned rooms or breezy outdoor places, may also be beneficial.

Light Sensitivity:

It is usual to have increased sensitivity to light following LASIK surgery. Wear sunglasses outside, particularly on bright or sunny days, to protect your eyes from glare and UV rays.

Limiting screen time and reducing interior illumination may also help alleviate pain.

Halos or glare:

Some patients who have had LASIK surgery may perceive halos or glare near lights, especially at night. This side effect normally goes away on its own as your eyes recover, but if it continues or worsens over time, contact your surgeon for additional assessment.

Discomfort:

If you have chronic or severe discomfort, such as pain, redness, or impaired vision, call your eye surgeon right away. These might be indications of issues that need immediate care.

Follow-Up Appointments And Long-Term Care

Regular follow-up appointments with your eye surgeon are vital for tracking your development and assuring the best possible results following LASIK surgery. Here's what you may anticipate throughout these appointments:

First Post-Operation Visit:

Your initial follow-up visit will normally take place the day following your operation. During this appointment, your surgeon will inspect your eyes for symptoms of problems and offer further post-operative advice.

Subsequent visits:

You will most likely have further follow-up visits in the weeks and months after your LASIK procedure. These appointments enable your surgeon to check on your healing process, evaluate your vision, and address any concerns you may have.

Long-term Care:
Even after your eyes have completely recovered, you should schedule frequent eye examinations with your optometrist or ophthalmologist to check your vision

and general eye health. While LASIK surgery may treat a variety of vision disorders, it is not a permanent cure, and your eyesight may change over time.

By following your surgeon's post-operative care recommendations and attending frequent follow-up visits, you may ensure the best possible results and have a clear vision for years to come.

CHAPTER 7

Risks And Complications

Common Dangers Related To LASIK

LASIK, like any surgical treatment, has certain hazards. While it is usually regarded as safe and successful, there are certain risks that patients should be aware of before having the treatment.

One typical danger is dry eyes. After LASIK, some patients may suffer dryness, which may be uncomfortable and impair visual quality. This happens because the procedure may affect the nerves that control tear production. However, this is often transient and may be treated with lubricating eye drops.

Another concern is over- or under-correction of eyesight. While developments in LASIK technology have considerably decreased the probability of this occurring, it remains a possibility. Overcorrection occurs when too much tissue is removed from the cornea, resulting in sharper vision than desired. In contrast, under-correction occurs when insufficient tissue is removed, necessitating the continuing use of glasses or contact lenses.

Flap problems are also conceivable with LASIK surgery. The corneal flap formed after the operation may not adhere adequately or get dislodged, resulting in problems like as infection or uneven astigmatism. However, these events are uncommon and may typically be resolved with further therapy.

Potential Issues And How They Are Handled

In addition to the dangers outlined above, various issues might occur during or after LASIK surgery. This includes:

1. **Infection:** Although LASIK is done in a sterile setting to reduce the risk of infection, it may still occur. Infection symptoms may include redness, discomfort, and ocular discharge. If an infection is detected, get early medical assistance to avoid consequences.

2. **Glare or halos:** Some patients may notice glare or halos near lights, particularly at night. This may impair night vision, and it may be particularly noticeable in people with bigger pupils. These symptoms usually resolve with time as the eyes recover, but in rare situations, extra therapy may be required.

3. Corneal ectasia is an uncommon but significant condition in which the cornea weakens and bulges outward, resulting in a gradual loss of eyesight. Patients with thin corneas or other risk factors may be more vulnerable to this condition. In extreme circumstances, a cornea transplant may be required to restore eyesight.

4. **Regression:** Some individuals may have regression, which is when their eyesight progressively declines following LASIK surgery. This might be caused by natural changes in the eye or other things. In such circumstances, boosts or retreatments may be advised to provide good vision.

Long-Term Hazards And Uncommon Consequences

While LASIK is generally regarded as a safe and successful operation for the majority of patients, there are certain long-term concerns and uncommon problems to consider. This includes:

1. **Dry eye syndrome:** In certain situations, dry eye symptoms may last a long time following LASIK surgery, necessitating continuing therapy with lubricating eye drops or other therapies.

2. **Vision changes:** Although LASIK may correct refractive defects such as nearsightedness,

farsightedness, and astigmatism, it cannot prevent age-related vision changes like presbyopia. As patients mature, they may still need reading glasses or other vision correction choices.

3. **Corneal thinning:** LASIK is a procedure that removes corneal tissue to reshape the cornea and improve eyesight. In rare circumstances, this might result in gradual thinning of the cornea over time, thereby raising the risk of issues including corneal ectasia.

4. **Complications of enhancement operations:** In certain situations, patients may need to undergo further surgeries, known as enhancements or retreatments, to obtain the required visual correction. While these operations are typically safe, they pose risks comparable to the first LASIK surgery.

How To Reduce Risks And Achieve A Favorable Result

While LASIK surgery does have certain hazards, some procedures may be done to reduce these risks and ensure a healthy result. This includes:

1. Choosing a competent physician: One of the most crucial aspects of guaranteeing a successful LASIK procedure is hiring a professional and experienced surgeon. Patients should do comprehensive research on possible surgeons, taking into account qualifications, expertise, and patient satisfaction ratings.

2. Following pre-operative instructions: Before LASIK surgery, patients will be given detailed directions by their surgeon on how to prepare for the process. This might involve avoiding contact lenses, stopping some drugs, and refraining from drinking and smoking. Following these recommendations properly may help lessen the likelihood of problems after surgery.

3. Disclosing medical history and risk factors: Patients should reveal their whole medical history to their surgeon, including any pre-existing eye diseases, drugs, or allergies. Certain conditions, including as thin corneas or autoimmune illnesses, might increase the risk of problems and should be addressed with the physician before surgery.

4. Awareness of the technique and the dangers: Before having LASIK surgery, patients should have a complete awareness of the operation, as well as the risks and issues that may arise. This involves considering alternate treatment choices and setting realistic expectations for vision repair.

5. After LASIK surgery, patients will be given particular post-operative care recommendations, such as using prescribed eye drops, avoiding vigorous activities, and attending follow-up visits with their physician. Adherence to these directions is critical for good healing and reducing the risk of problems.

Patients who take these measures and work closely with a trained surgeon may reduce the dangers of LASIK surgery and boost their chances of success. However, no surgical treatment is without risk, and patients should carefully consider the possible advantages and downsides before making a choice.

CHAPTER 8

Alternatives To Lasik

Other Refractive Surgeries

When contemplating vision correction surgery, LASIK is not the only choice. Other techniques include photorefractive keratectomy (PRK), laser epithelial keratomileusis (LASEK), and small incision lenticule extraction (SMILE). These operations follow similar concepts to LASIK but may vary in methodology and appropriateness for certain people.

PRK involves reshaping the cornea using an excimer laser, similar to LASIK. Instead of forming a flap in the cornea, the surgeon removes the outer layer (epithelium) before altering the underlying tissue. PRK is often indicated for individuals who have thin corneas or other corneal abnormalities that render LASIK ineffective.

LASEK is similar to PRK in that it preserves a small layer of the epithelium, which is then restored after the cornea is reshaped. This may cause less pain during recovery than PRK, but it may also take longer to heal.

SMILE: SMILE is a newer method for correcting eyesight by reshaping the cornea. Instead of using a laser to make a flap or remove the epithelium, SMILE involves making a tiny incision in the cornea and removing a lenticular (a small piece of corneal tissue), which alters the curvature of the cornea. SMILE is generally favored since it is less intrusive and may result in a speedier recovery.

Each of these techniques has its own set of benefits and concerns. For example, although LASIK usually provides faster visual recovery than PRK or LASEK, PRK may be a preferable choice for those with certain corneal features. SMILE, on the other hand, may appeal to people who are worried about the formation of a corneal flap.

Nonsurgical Options

Non-surgical methods such as glasses and contact lenses remain feasible for people who choose not to undergo surgery or are ineligible for refractive surgery. Glasses are a simple and non-invasive technique to correct eyesight, and contemporary lens technologies allow a variety of solutions to accommodate varied prescriptions and lifestyle preferences.

Contact lenses, whether soft or hard gas permeable, provide an additional non-surgical alternative for vision correction. Contact lenses provide the extra advantage of not affecting one's look, as glasses do, and may give superior peripheral vision. Contact lenses, on the other hand, need frequent care and may not be appropriate for everyone, especially those with certain eye diseases or lifestyle choices.

Comparing LASIK To Other Vision Correction Methods

When comparing LASIK to alternative vision correction techniques, various criteria are taken into account, including efficacy, safety, convenience, and cost. LASIK is often recommended for its rapid recovery period and high success rate, however, it may not be the best choice for everyone. PRK, LASEK, and SMILE are options that may be better suited for people with certain eye traits or preferences.

Glasses and contact lenses, although non-surgical, offer adequate vision correction for many individuals and may be chosen for their convenience and versatility. However, they need continuing care and may not give permanent correction, as refractive surgery does.

Choosing The Best Option For Your Needs

Ultimately, the ideal vision correction solution for you is determined by a variety of criteria, including your eye health, prescription, lifestyle, preferences, and budget. It is important to contact an expert eye care practitioner who can evaluate your unique requirements and propose the best treatment choice.

During your appointment, your eye doctor will assess your eye health, measure your prescription, and talk about your objectives and concerns. They will then provide specialized suggestions based on your specific condition, including LASIK, alternative refractive surgery, and non-surgical treatments like as glasses or contact lenses.

You can make an educated choice about the best technique to get a clear and comfortable vision by balancing the benefits and drawbacks of each option and taking into account your specific requirements.

Remember that vision correction is a big investment in your quality of life, so research your alternatives extensively and choose the solution that best meets your requirements and preferences.

CHAPTER 9

Cost And Insurance Considerations

Typical Prices For LASIK Surgery

Understanding the normal expenses of LASIK surgery is critical for anybody contemplating the treatment. The cost varies based on numerous aspects, such as the technology utilized, the surgeon's skill, and the clinic's location.

The typical cost of LASIK surgery in the United States is between $2,000 and $3,000 per eye. However, it is important to remember that this is just an estimate, and real prices may differ. Some clinics may charge less, while others may charge more, particularly if they utilize innovative equipment or employ highly skilled surgeons.

When comparing prices at various clinics, it is important to examine what is included in the pricing. Some clinics may provide a cheaper initial fee but charge more for pre-operative consultations, post-operative care, or improvements. On the other hand, certain clinics may provide an all-inclusive package that includes everything from the first consultation to follow-up sessions.

It's also vital to ask about any possible hidden fees or extra expenditures that may develop during or after the procedure. These may include fees for drugs, upgrades, or post-operative care. Understanding the entire range of expenses connected with LASIK surgery allows you to make a better-educated choice about whether it is the best option for you.

Factors That Impact Costs

The cost of LASIK surgery may be influenced by a variety of variables, including the technology employed, the surgeon's expertise, and clinic location.

The technologies employed during the treatment might significantly affect the cost. Advanced LASIK technologies, including bladeless LASIK or wavefront-guided LASIK, may be more expensive than regular LASIK procedures. These technologies provide more accuracy and perhaps better results, but they frequently come at a larger cost.

The surgeon's skill and reputation might influence the cost of LASIK surgery. Surgeons with greater expertise and a track record of successful treatments may charge more for their services. However, it is important to realize that the cost of LASIK surgery should not be the only consideration when selecting a specialist. Quality and safety should always be a top priority.

Furthermore, the location of the facility might affect the cost of LASIK treatment. Clinics in big urban regions or wealthy communities may charge greater rates than those in rural or less affluent locations. However, considerations other than cost should be considered, such as the clinic's reputation and the quality of treatment delivered.

Insurance Coverage And Financing Alternatives

Many health insurance companies exclude LASIK surgery because it is considered an elective operation. However, some insurance companies provide discounts or reimbursement for LASIK procedures as part of a vision care package. Check with your insurance provider to determine whether the LASIK procedure is covered by your plan and if there are any discounts or reimbursement alternatives available.

If your insurance does not cover LASIK surgery, there are financing alternatives available to assist you pay the treatment. Many LASIK clinics have financing solutions that include cheap monthly payments and free or moderate interest rates. Furthermore, some third-party financing organizations specialize in medical treatments such as LASIK surgery, providing reasonable rates and flexible payback options.

Before agreeing to a financing plan, thoroughly read the terms and conditions, including any interest rates, fees, or penalties for late payments. It is also critical to assess your budget and financial condition to ensure that you can easily make the monthly payments.

How To Analyze And Choose A LASIK Provider

Choosing the correct LASIK provider is critical for getting the best possible results from your procedure. When considering LASIK providers, consider the following factors:

1. Experience and expertise: Look into the credentials and experience of the surgeon who will conduct your LASIK procedure. Look for a board-certified surgeon with substantial expertise in conducting LASIK treatments.

2. Inquire about the technology and equipment utilized at the LASIK clinic. Choose a provider that uses cutting-edge, FDA-approved technology to get the greatest outcomes.

3. **Reputation and reviews:** Read reviews and testimonials from former patients to have an understanding of the clinic's reputation and the level of treatment offered. Look for a practitioner with a history of positive results and delighted patients.

4. **Appointment process:** Set up an appointment with the LASIK specialist to discuss your candidacy for the treatment and ask any questions you may have. Pay attention to how the employees treat you and if they take the time to answer your problems.

5. Consider the cost of LASIK surgery and any financing alternatives. Choose a supplier that provides upfront pricing and flexible payment options to make the operation more affordable.

By carefully examining these variables and selecting a trustworthy LASIK provider, you may boost your chances of having a successful procedure. Don't be afraid to ask questions and get several viewpoints before making a choice. Your eyesight is valuable, so find a provider you can trust to give the finest possible treatment.

CHAPTER 10

Advancements In LASIK Technology

Latest Innovations In LASIK Technology

The world of LASIK technology is continually changing, with developments pushing the limits of what is possible in vision repair. One of the most interesting advancements is the advent of bladeless LASIK, which substitutes the standard microkeratome blade with a femtosecond laser to create the corneal flap. This improves accuracy while lowering the risk of problems associated with blade usage.

Another innovation is the use of wavefront technology in LASIK operations. This enables a tailored treatment strategy based on the unique features of each person's eyes. Wavefront-guided LASIK achieves improved levels of visual acuity while reducing the incidence of side effects such as glare and halos by mapping the complete optical pathway, including any aberrations or defects.

Furthermore, advances in excimer laser technology have resulted in the creation of quicker and more accurate laser systems. This implies shorter treatment durations and better results for people having LASIK surgery. Furthermore, eye-tracking technology keeps the laser properly aligned with the eye's motions, increasing safety and precision.

Custom LASIK And Wavefront-Guided Procedures

Custom LASIK takes tailored vision correction to the next level by using new diagnostic techniques to assess each patient's unique eye features. Custom LASIK provides a specific treatment plan by assessing characteristics such as corneal shape, pupil size, and refractive errors, resulting in better visual results and lower risk of problems.

Wavefront-guided treatments expand on this personalization by employing extensive measurements of the eye's optical system to direct the laser in reshaping the cornea. This corrects not just refractive problems like nearsightedness, farsightedness, and astigmatism, but also higher-order aberrations that may degrade visual quality. By carefully correcting these flaws, wavefront-guided LASIK allows patients to have sharper, clearer vision with fewer visual disruptions.

These new technologies represent a substantial advancement in refractive surgery, providing patients with unparalleled levels of accuracy, safety, and customization. As technology advances, we may anticipate more modifications and breakthroughs that will improve the LASIK experience and broaden the options for vision correction.

The Future Of LASIK: Emerging Trends

Looking forward, the future of LASIK offers opportunities for continuous innovation and refining of current technology. One area of continuing study is the creation of new laser systems with even higher levels of accuracy and efficiency. Researchers want to enhance results and broaden the spectrum of curable refractive defects by using femtosecond lasers and other cutting-edge technology.

Furthermore, advances in artificial intelligence and machine learning are expected to transform the area of refractive surgery. These technologies can analyze massive volumes of data to uncover patterns and trends that may guide tailored treatment strategies and improve surgical results. Using AI-powered algorithms, doctors may be able to attain even better levels of precision and predictability in LASIK treatments.

Furthermore, current advancements in LASIK surgery include the development of less invasive procedures that decrease corneal stress and speed up recovery time. These procedures attempt to make LASIK surgery more accessible to a broader variety of patients, including those with thin or uneven corneas who were previously unsuitable for classic LASIK.

Overall, the future of LASIK seems promising, with advances in technology and technique driving improvements in safety, effectiveness, and patient satisfaction. As academics and doctors work together to push the limits of what is possible in vision correction, LASIK surgery is expected to stay at the forefront of refractive surgery for many years to come.

How Technology Improves Results And Safety

The use of sophisticated technologies in LASIK operations has considerably improved both surgical results and patient safety.

By improving treatment accuracy, predictability, and customization, technology enables surgeons to perform more precise refractive repairs with fewer problems.

For example, using femtosecond lasers to create flaps minimizes the risk of flap-related problems such as uneven flap margins, buttonholes, and epithelial ingrowth. Similarly, bespoke LASIK and wavefront-guided treatments allow doctors to correct not just fundamental refractive errors, but also secondary aberrations that may impair visual quality and clarity.

Furthermore, advances in diagnostic imaging and biomechanical analysis have improved pre-operative screening processes, enabling surgeons to identify and categorize patients based on their risk profile and appropriateness for LASIK. This proactive strategy reduces the number of adverse events and guarantees that patients only get surgery if they are likely to benefit from it.

Overall, the incorporation of cutting-edge technology into LASIK surgery has elevated the operation from a one-size-fits-all to a highly individualized and precise treatment choice. By using the most recent advances in laser technology, imaging technologies, and data analytics, LASIK surgeons can provide patients with unsurpassed visual results and safety, paving the way for a future in which refractive defects are readily corrected and vision is maximized for everyone.

Conclusion

Finally, reading the Complete Guide to Grasp LASIK Eye Surgery provides a comprehensive grasp of this transforming surgery. LASIK (Laser-Assisted In Situ Keratomileusis) has become the gold standard for vision correction, allowing people to break free from the constraints of glasses or contacts. A thorough examination of the process, its advantages, hazards, and developments reveals numerous crucial truths.

First and foremost, LASIK surgery is an amazing combination of cutting-edge technology and medical competence. Laser technology's precision enables extraordinary corneal reshaping, allowing patients to attain amazing visual acuity. This technical capability, along with surgeons' expertise and experience, assures that the treatment is safe and effective.

Furthermore, the advantages of LASIK go well beyond optical clarity. For many people, LASIK offers newfound freedom - freedom from the hassle of corrective glasses, freedom to participate in activities without restriction, and freedom to explore the world without visual constraints. This improved quality of life is one of the most significant benefits of LASIK surgery, allowing people to fully enjoy life's events with confidence and clarity.

However, it is critical to recognize that LASIK surgery, like other medical procedures, has inherent dangers and restrictions. While technological and surgical breakthroughs have considerably reduced these dangers, problems like as dry eyes, glare, halos, and under or overcorrection are still possible. Thus, informed consent and a comprehensive preoperative examination are critical components of the LASIK procedure, ensuring that patients have reasonable expectations and understand the possible results.

Furthermore, the LASIK surgical scene is always evolving, with continual research and development pushing the limits of what is feasible. From advances in laser technology to revolutionary surgical procedures, the future of vision correction promises even more accuracy, safety, and customization.

Ultimately, the choice to get LASIK surgery is extremely personal, impacted by individual circumstances, tastes, and expectations. While the Complete Guide to Understanding LASIK Eye Surgery provides comprehensive knowledge and insights, prospective patients should have an open dialogue with their eye care providers, asking questions, expressing concerns, and weighing the risks and benefits before making a decision.

In essence, LASIK surgery represents the junction of science, technology, and human inventiveness, providing a game-changing option for vision correction. Individuals who embrace a comprehensive knowledge of the treatment may begin on their LASIK journey with confidence, knowing that they are equipped to make educated choices regarding their eye health and visual well-being.

THE END

www.ingramcontent.com/pod-product-compliance
Lightning Source LLC
Chambersburg PA
CBHW071837210526
45479CB00001B/181